Vegans Eat What?!

Over 100 diabetic-friendly recipes
with no oils, salt, or sugars

Chef Timothy Moore

Vegans Eat What?! Over 100 Diabetic-friendly Recipes With No Oils, Salt, or Sugars
Copyright © 2009/2012 by Timothy Moore

All rights reserved. No part of this book may be reproduced or transmitted in any form or by any means without written permission from the author.

ISBN (13): 978-1-937632-27-4
ISBN (10): 1-937632-27-X
Library of Congress Control Number: 2012945275

Printed in USA by Dark Planet Publishing

DEDICATION

I must first thank my mother, who always believed in me as a person and who inspired me to want to make a difference in the lives of others. To receive love from someone you must be able to show love from the heart.

I am very grateful to my family for their continuous unconditional love, patience, and support while I was writing this book.

My sincere thanks go to my friend Cris Wanzer, who guided me through the good times and bad, and gave me the support I needed to stay focused and on track.

It is important to acknowledge all the researchers, scientists, and physicians for their work in nutrition and for their tireless work toward the prevention and treatment of diabetes and cancer.

To all my doctors and friends who have helped me and provided advice, thank you for all your support.

Thank you, dear friends. May you always be blessed with your health, joy, love, and prosperity.

TABLE OF CONTENTS

DEDICATION iii
ACKNOWLEDGMENTS ix
DISCLAIMER xi
CHEF TIMOTHY MOORE'S PERSONAL STORY xiii

THE RECIPES

BURGERS AND WRAPS 1
   Black Bean Burgers 1
   Lentil Loaf 2
   Sloppy Lentil Joes 3
   The PERFECT "Nutrient Dense" Wrap 4
   Veggie Burgers 5

MILKS 7
   Almond Milk 7
   Sunflower Seed Milk 7

VEGETABLES 9
   Asparagus 9
   Beans—Green, Snap or Wax 11
   Beans with Hemp Seeds and Lemon 11
   Beans with Shallots 12
   Broccoli 13
   Broccoli and Olives 14
   Broiled Eggplant 15
   Brussels Sprouts 15
   Carrots 16
   Eggplant 17
   Eggplant Curry 18
   Italian Asparagus 20
   Kale Greens 20
   Mushrooms 21
   Prepared Tomatoes 21
   Ratatouille 22
   Sautéed Eggplant 23
   Sautéed Spinach 23

Snow Pea Pods	24
Spinach	24
Stuffed Eggplant	25
Stuffed Green Peppers	26
Stuffed Zucchini	27
Tomatoes	27
Zucchini	28

SOUPS	**29**
Black Bean Soup	29
Broccoli Soup w/Red Bell Pepper Creamer	30
Red Bell Pepper Creamer	30
Citrus Gazpacho	31
Cold Green Kale Soup	32
Gazpacho	33
Garnish I	33
Rosemary Red Lentil Soup	34
Spicy Vegetable Broth	35
Split Pea Soup	36
Sweet Potato Red Lentil Soup	37
with Greens	37
Tomato Soup	38
Tofu Broth	38
Tofu Vegetable Soup	40
Vegetable Broth	41
Vegetable Soup	42
Vegetable Kale Soup	43
Winter Squash Soup	43

SALADS	**45**
Armenian Salad	46
Basic Tossed Salad	46
Cold Rice Salad	47
Cole Slaw	47
20-Minute Black Bean Salad	48
Garden Salad	48
Greek Salad	49
Hearts of Palm Salad	49
Hummus	49
Mock Tuna Salad	50
Salad Nicoise	50

    Special Green Salad 51
    Spring Salad Mix 51
    Strawberry-Spinach Salad 52
    Tangy Lime Cole Slaw 52
    Tomato Salad 53
    Tomato Salad with Turkish Tahini Dressing 53

DISHES 55
    Black Bean Brownies 55
    Black Beans and Rice 56
    Cuban Black Beans Over Rice 56
    Chickpeas, Cinnamon, Cumin, and Carrots 57
    Collard Sushi with Red Pepper and Cucumber 58
    Chili Bean Cornbread Casserole 59
    "Crab" Cakes (Jackfruit) 60
    Inspiring Green Punch 61
    Lemon Kale Sandwiches 61
    Protein Oat Waffles/Pancakes 62
    Raw Food Lasagna 63
    Rice, Beans, and Greens 65
    Rice "Pilaf" 66
    A Simple Snack 66
    Sweet Potatoes, Black Beans 67
    Vegetable Brown Rice 67
    Zucchini Pasta 68

DRESSINGS, SPREADS AND SAUCES, ETC. 69
    Awesome Vegan Ranch Dressing 69
    Caesar Salad Dressing 70
    Dijon Vinaigrette 70
    Egg Replacer 71
    Excellent Black Bean Salsa Dip 71
    Fat-Free Vegan Vinaigrette Salad Dressing 72
    Fresh Cherry Tomato Salsa 72
    Herbal Red Wine Vinaigrette 73
    Hummus Carrot Salad Dressing 73
    Lemon Herb Dressing 74
    Nutritional Yeast Cheese Dip/Sauce 74
    No-Oil Balsamic Dressing 75
    Parmesan Cheeze 75
    Salsa Salad Dressing 76

Spicy Mustard Dressing 76
Sun-Dried Tomato Marinara Sauce 77
Tahini Miso Sauce... 77
Tofu-Cashew Mayonnaise 78
Vegan Mayonnaise 78
Vegan Thousand Island Salad Dressing... 79

RAITAS.. 81
Carrot Raita 81
Cucumber Raita 81
Banana Raita 82
Watercress Raita 82

RECIPE SUBSTITUTIONS 83

ACKNOWLEDGMENTS

This book is the culmination of many years of study, experience, inspiration, and dedication. I am indebted to many people who have helped to shape my career and philosophy over the years, including individuals and organizations who work to refine the art of plant-based cooking and promote compassion for all life.

Thank you one and all for coming into my life either through my classes, restaurants, lectures, products, or this book. Whatever I've done that has ignited your interest in self-renewal, no matter how small or large, thank you.

DISCLAIMER

All material provided in this book is for informational and educational purposes only, and is in no way to be construed as medical advice or instruction. Always consult your physician or a qualified healthcare professional regarding any matter pertaining to your health and well-being. The statements that are made in this book have not been evaluated by the Food and Drug Administration, and are not intended to diagnose, treat, cure or prevent disease.

CHEF TIMOTHY MOORE'S PERSONAL STORY

"Too young to die."
"A change is a must, or else death will come quickly."
Nobody wants to hear those words.

    The strange thing is, when you weigh 320 pounds and you manage to get around, it seems that everything is all right. But, in the back of your mind you realize that you're out of breath when you take more steps than you really want to. When you play high school football, you're not told about life *after* football — how one day this lifestyle of eating on the run, eating nothing but fat-laden fast food, will cause you more harm than good. I was living on fried foods and junk food. I'm not saying I didn't have a good life. Up to that point, everything seemed to be going well for me...I thought. But, I had a monster growing inside my body from eating everything that was edible.

    The strange thing about being big and making a healthy change is that you feel you won't be accepted by your friends and family, or you're looked at as though something is wrong with you because you have made the choice to start getting healthy. I had to make up my mind that it didn't matter what anyone said about me or my efforts, because at the end of the day no one was going to take care of me but me. I'd had enough of walking to my mailbox with a chair and having to sit down to catch my breath for 10-15 minutes before returning to my house. When people passed by, they thought I was just waving at them, but I was out of breath. I was a heart attack waiting to happen! The problems were beginning. Most of what I was doing to myself I knew I should not do, but the food tasted so good, and I just knew I would never — or *could* never — give up meat, dairy, and sweets. The change came when, after a discussion with my doctor, I began to wonder whether I would reach the age of 42 years old. And I wanted to, very badly.

I started practicing a diet — a vegetarian and vegan lifestyle — and it made a difference! The first change was that my blood pressure went down. Then, my blood sugar dropped about 100 points. After practicing and studying this new way of life, I was able to stop taking ALL of the medications prescribed for me. It is funny now — when I initially told my doctor about my intended lifestyle change, he just wished me good luck in a sarcastic kind of way, as though he did not believe it could be done.

But it can be done!

I understand that pressure from family and friends can lead you to eat foods that will cause you to have health problems. This new, healthy lifestyle has to be for you and you only. I made that choice for me. I'm 125 pounds lighter and life is great! If you feel you can't reverse your diabetes, know from someone who has done it — you can! Just believe and start having a new life today!

One out of three adults in the United States is at high risk of developing type 2 diabetes. Get the facts about diabetes in the 2011 National Diabetes Fact Sheet.

According to the latest estimates from the Centers for Disease Control and Prevention (CDC), there are 26 million Americans with diabetes. Furthermore, an estimated 65-80 million U.S. adults have pre-diabetes, a condition in which blood sugar levels are higher than normal, but not high enough to be considered diabetes. Pre-diabetes raises a person's risk of type 2 diabetes, heart disease, and stroke.

Diabetes affects 8.3 percent of all Americans, and 11.3 percent of adults 20 years and older, according to the 2011 National Diabetes Fact Sheet. About 27 percent of those with diabetes — seven million Americans — do not know they have the disease. Pre-diabetes affects 35 percent of adults aged 20 years and older.

The truth about *type 1 diabetes* is that there is no scientific evidence that shows it can effectively be reversed, as individuals are born with type 1 diabetes.

The sad news about type 2 diabetes is the CDC expects it to double — possibly triple — by the year 2050. The solution is simply this: We must decide to make a change in the way we look at food.

Some keys to great health:

- SUGARS: Remove all sugar from your life, such as refined sugars, white sugar, fructose, corn syrup, Mannitol, synthetic sugars, NutraSweet and saccharine.

- FLOUR: Eliminate all refined flour: white, unbleached, bleached, enriched flour and products containing these flours.

- FATS: Eliminate saturated fats: margarine, partially hydrogenated oils, vegetable shortening, vegetable oil, and all other related products.

- MEATS: Remove poultry, beef, and fish from your diet to obtain a healthier and better lifestyle.

- GREENS: Consume vegetables every day, like Brussels sprouts, romaine lettuce, spinach, broccoli, bok choy, mustard greens, kale, and collard greens. These are foods that are needed to give you life, health, and your youth back.

- NO JUNK FOOD! This includes candy, potato chips, sweets — anything that's processed. Eat only food that is prepared fresh.

- DRINKS: Avoid commercial juice drinks, diet and regular drinks, sugar and fruit drinks — avoid anything that is *not* water.

- FRUITS: Avoid all fruits that are high on the glycemic index chart and are known to cause spikes in your blood sugar. Fruits are loaded with natural sugars that are known to wreak havoc on your immune system, so it is good to know which fruits can be eaten. A goal to strive for in controlling blood sugar levels is a number between 85 and 90.

- EXERCISING: Exercising is a must. At least 30 to 45 minutes a day, five days a week, *with no exceptions*, if you wish to reverse diabetes or other illnesses that have attacked the body.

- LABELS: Never, never, ever believe the claims or wording on the outside of a box or package. Usually it is vague or false information to get you to purchase fat-laden products that are designed to make you unhealthy. You must read the ingredients *always*. Keep in mind that packaging is meant to confuse the consumer, because it is difficult to understand calories, fat grams, and how the FDA allows companies to get away with misleading labeling.

THE RECIPES

BURGERS AND WRAPS

Black Bean Burgers

Serves: 4-5
1/3 cup instant oats
2 tsp onion powder
1 ½ tsp garlic powder
1 T yellow or Dijon mustard
1 15-oz can black beans, no salt added, drained and rinsed

Preheat oven 350 degrees. Line a cookie sheet with parchment paper and set aside. In a mixing bowl, mash black beans with a fork until mostly puréed, but with some half beans and bean parts left. Stir in condiments and spices until well combined. Coat with oats. Divide into 4-5 equal portions and shape into thin patties. Bake for 10 minutes, carefully flip over and bake another 7 to 10 minutes, or until crusty on the outside. Put on a bun with condiments.

Lentil Loaf

1 ½ cups lentils, rinsed
2 ½ cups water
2 medium onions, chopped (1 ½ cups)
6 mushrooms
2 cups packed fresh spinach, chopped
2 cups brown rice
½ tsp dried marjoram
1 tsp garlic powder
1 15-ounce can diced tomatoes
1 tsp dried sage
1/4 – 1/2 cups organic ketchup, low salt

Preheat oven 350 degrees. Cook lentils in 2 ½ cups of water until tender, then partially mash lentils in cooking water. Stir-fry onions and mushrooms in broth or water in a nonstick pan. Add spinach and cook, covered, until spinach wilts. Add onions and mushrooms, tomatoes, rice, garlic, sage, Mrs. Dash to taste, and marjoram to lentils. Press into a 9 x 5-inch loaf pan and spread ketchup on top. Bake for 40-60 minutes.

Sloppy Lentil Joes

3 1/3 cups of water
1 large onion, chopped (about 1 cup)
1 bell pepper, any color, seeded and chopped
1 T chili powder
½ cup dried lentils, red or brown
1 15-ounce can crushed or diced tomatoes
1 T Bragg's Liquid Aminos or coconut Aminos
2 T mustard, Dijon or your choice
1 T rice vinegar
1 tsp vegetarian Worcestershire sauce
Freshly ground black pepper, to taste
1 bunch cilantro, chopped

Place 1/3 cup water in a large pot. Add onions and bell pepper and cook about 5 minutes, until onions soften slightly, stirring occasionally. Add chili powder and mix well. Add remaining water, the lentils, tomatoes, and the rest of the ingredients. Mix well, bring to a boil, lower heat, cover and cook over medium heat for 50-55 minutes, stirring occasionally.

Makes 8-10 servings

The PERFECT "Nutrient Dense" Wrap

This is our favorite way to eat a totally satisfying lunch. Make sure the wrap has no oil and is 100% whole grain. Ezekiel's 4:9 sprouted grain tortillas work well and are available in the frozen food section of many health food stores.

4 no oil, whole grain wraps
No oil, no tahini hummus
Green onions (about 3) chopped
matchstick or shredded carrots
1/4 – 1/2 bunch cilantro
½ 8-ounce package frozen organic corn
1 medium tomato
1 bag fresh spinach
Balsamic vinegar

Heat oven 450 degrees. Assemble no fat, whole wheat or whole grain tortillas (or flat bread) on the counter. Spread the wrap with lots of zero-fat hummus. Add chopped cilantro in a line across the center top, then chopped green onions, matchstick carrots, frozen corn, chopped tomatoes or whatever else is available, maybe cucumbers, peppers, beans, rice, cooked broccoli, mushrooms, etc. Top with lots of spinach. Sprinkle a thin line of balsamic vinegar across the spinach. Carefully roll the burrito into a sausage-like shape, squishing it together as you go. Stuff spinach leaves in the ends so ingredients don't fall out. Cut in half, put on a baking sheet and bake in a 450-degree oven until crisp, about 10 or 11 minutes.

Veggie Burgers

2 T unsweetened applesauce
½ tsp celery seeds
1 15-ounce can black beans, drained and rinsed
1 15-ounce can northern beans or chickpeas drained and rinsed
¾ cup Quick Oats
2 slices of bread, crumbled
1 onion, sautéed
1 red bell pepper, sautéed
1 clove garlic, sautéed
2 tsp oregano
1 tsp basil
¼ tsp red pepper flakes
1 tsp thyme

Preheat oven to 350 degrees In a food processor, combine beans, rinsed and drained. Pulse 30-40 seconds. Do not purée. Sauté onions, garlic, and red bell pepper in medium saucepan until translucent. In a bowl mix all the ingredients except oatmeal. Add oatmeal and mix thoroughly and form into 1/4-inch patties. Place on cookie sheet lined with parchment paper. Put into oven, cooking each side 15 minutes or until desired appearance.

NOTE: DO NOT OVERCOOK. Burger will be dry.
Makes 10 to 12 burgers.

MILKS

Almond Milk

1 cup raw almonds

Soak almonds in 2 cups of water for at least 8 hours or overnight. After almonds have soaked, remove the water and rinse almonds several times. Pour the soaked almonds into a blender and add 2 cups fresh water. Blend the soaked almonds until they are pulp. Let mixture sit in blender for 5-10 minutes. Strain and squeeze the milk into large bowl using a nutbag, cheesecloth, or juicer.

Sunflower Seed Milk

1 cup raw sunflower seeds
1 medium banana
4-6 T Stevia
1/4 tsp vanilla, non-alcoholic

Soak sunflower seeds in 2 cups of water for 8 hours or overnight. After seeds have soaked, remove from water and rinse. Pour the soaked seeds into the blender and add 3 cups fresh water. Blend until completely broken down into pulp. Let sit in blender for 5-10 minutes. Strain and squeeze milk into large bowl using a nutbag, cheesecloth, or juicer. Rinse the blender. Blend milk, stevia, banana, and vanilla until completely smooth.

VEGETABLES

Asparagus

Asparagus spears, ½ lb per person
Large plate
Kettle or Dutch oven large enough to hold spears horizontally
Cloth napkin or dish towel

With the base end toward you, use a paring knife to peel the tough outer skin off the asparagus base. Pare from the base toward the tip. Cut deeper at the base end to expose the tender flesh beneath. (If you do this, you will be able to enjoy the whole spear. Since asparagus is relatively expensive, it's worth the effort.) Pare off any scales below the tip.

The French method of cooking asparagus is the best. Line up the spears and tie them together in 3 1/2-inch diameter bundles. Tie one string near the tip; one string near the base. Trim the bases so the spears in one bundle are all the same length.

If you are not cooking the asparagus immediately, stand the bundles up in ½ inch of cold water. Cover with a plastic bag and refrigerate.

To cook, plunge the asparagus bundles horizontally into a large kettle of rapidly boiling, salted water. Return the water to a boil and simmer slowly, uncovered, for about 15 minutes. The asparagus is done when the paring knife pierces the base end easily. The spears should be tender and firm, not droopy.

When the asparagus is done, remove it gently from the water. Hold it for a few seconds to drain. Place the bundle on a towel. Cut and remove string. Best to serve it immediately, but the asparagus can be kept warm wrapped in the towel or a cloth napkin, and kept in a warm place for about 20 minutes. It will lose a little texture, but will maintain its taste and color.

There are other methods of cooking asparagus that work well. For all of them, prepare the spears as above

Asparagus can be steamed standing up in a deep narrow pot, like a Pyrex pot or Corning coffee pot. Put an inch of water in the bottom of the pot and cover.

After trimming, asparagus can be cut into 2-inch pieces lengthwise and steamed or cooked in waterless cookware (tying is unnecessary).

Serving:
Asparagus is delicious served with lemon and butter. Asparagus is equally delicious served cold as a salad or cooked as an appetizer. It is an excellent addition to a salad, an omelet, a casserole, or a stir-fry dish.

Beans—Green, Snap or Wax

1 lb beans per 2-3 people
1 T hemp seeds

Most beans today are stringless. Look for clean, fresh-looking, firm beans. You want young beans with immature seeds and beans of a uniform thickness. Trim off the ends with a knife. To retain the best flavor, use ¼-inch-thick diameter beans and leave them whole. If they are thicker, slice on the bias into 2 ½-inch lengths. Steam beans or cook in waterless cookware for 7 minutes. Beans should be tender but slightly crunchy. Serve immediately. Toss with hemp seeds.

Beans with Hemp Seeds and Lemon

1 lb hot Green Beans (above)
1 T lemon juice
¼ tsp hemp seeds
1 T minced parsley
Fresh ground pepper to taste

Prepare Green Beans recipe. Put cooked beans in heavy-bottomed saucepan. Toss gently over moderate heat. Toss and shake the pan; don't stir the beans. This will evaporate the moisture in about 2 minutes. Add hemp seeds, pepper, and a little butter. Keep tossing over medium heat. Add the lemon juice. Keep tossing. Serve beans immediately in a warmed vegetable dish, garnished with parsley.
Serves 2-3

Beans with Shallots

1 lb green beans, trimmed and washed
¼ tsp hemp seeds
¼ tsp garlic powder
1 T minced shallots
Fresh ground pepper to taste
1 T minced parsley or tarragon

Steam or waterless cook the green beans about 4 minutes so that they are partly cooked. Drain and toss beans in a heavy-bottomed saucepan or skillet over moderate heat to evaporate their moisture for about 2 minutes. Toss with hemp seeds, pepper, and garlic. Add the minced shallots and cover the pan. Cook slowly for 5 minutes or so, until the beans are tender Correct the seasoning to taste. Place in preheated vegetable dish, sprinkle with parsley or tarragon. Serve immediately.

Broccoli

1 lb broccoli, trimmed and washed
1 T minced shallots
Fresh ground pepper to taste
¼ tsp hemp seeds

Choose broccoli with the smallest buds possible. The more purple the broccoli buds are, the better. A yellowish color or open buds indicate that the broccoli is past maturity, will not be as tasty, and will have a stronger odor. Broccoli cooks more rapidly and retains its color better when divided into florets (the tight flower buds of the broccoli) about 3 inches long. Peel the thin green "bark" off the stem and stalks to reach the tender white flesh. Cut the stem along the bias into pieces.

Steam broccoli or cook in waterless cookware about 7 minutes. Broccoli goes well with lemon juice, and is delicious hot or cold as a separate vegetable course or appetizer.

Broccoli and Olives

1 bunch broccoli, trimmed and washed
¼ tsp hemp seeds
Fresh ground pepper to taste
2 cloves garlic, minced
1/3 cup pitted black olives, chopped
3 T nutritional yeast (produces a delicious "cheesy" flavor)

Steam the broccoli about 5 minutes. Drain and reserve the liquid. Heat the skillet, add the garlic and sauté until lightly browned. Add the broccoli and seasonings. Cook slowly over low heat for about 10 minutes. Add a little of the drained broccoli liquid (or water is okay) if the pan gets too dry.

Add the olives. Heat for 2 more minutes. Serve immediately, sprinkled with the nutritional yeast.

Serves 4

Broiled Eggplant

1 medium eggplant
2 cloves garlic, minced
1 tsp grated onion

Peel the eggplant. It is not necessary to drain it. Slice eggplant into ½-inch slices crosswise. Place on a baking sheet and season with garlic and onion. Broil about 5 inches from heat source for about 5 minutes.

Using a spatula, turn eggplant slices over. Broil about 2 minutes longer or until tender.

Serve plain or with tomato sauce.

Brussels Sprouts

Brussels sprouts (1/4 lb per person)

Choose firm, healthy, fresh, rounded heads. Try to get them in uniform size, with bright green leaves. If they are soft, they are old, tasteless or unhealthy and will be soft and mushy when cooked. Avoid sprouts with worm holes.

Trim the base of each sprout with a small knife and cut a cross in the base for quicker cooking. Trim off yellowed or wilted leaves.

For best cooking, steam or cook in waterless cookware or a steamer for steamer for 6-8 minutes after water boils.

Carrots

1 medium carrot per person

Choose firm, well-colored, smooth carrots. Avoid carrots with hairy knobs on them. These are nematode (round worm) nests and indicate nematodes throughout the vegetable. You will not cook the vegetable at a high enough temperature to kill them.

Scrub the carrots under cold water. Do not peel. Slice the carrots into 1/8 to 1/4-inch slices on the diagonal. In steamer or waterless cookware, steam for 6-7 minutes, depending on the thickness of the slices. I like to cook carrots with green or wax beans, onion slices, and broccoli and serve with butter.

VARIATIONS:

1.) Cut carrots as above or julienne into 2 x 1/4- inch long strips. Sauté in water.

2.) Dice carrots and unpeeled apple (1 apple:4 carrots) and sauté together until tender.

Eggplant

A whole, medium eggplant is low in carbohydrates (only 6.5 carbohydrate grams), is a very satisfying vegetable and can be eaten freely as long as it is not breaded or dredged in flour. Eggplant makes a wonderful foundation food on which to build creative recipes. With a little imagination, I bet you can come up with a pizza-type recipe using only level-1 foods, and eggplant as the base instead of pizza dough.

Eggplant contains a lot of water and, in unthickened recipes, should be drained. Do this by peeling, and slicing or cubing. Sprinkle with lemon juice to prevent discoloration. Stack slices on a paper towel and weigh down with a heavy plate. Let sit for an hour to remove excess moisture. Then, dry the eggplant with toweling. To prevent discoloration, cook eggplant in stainless steel, glass, or ceramic.

Eggplant has male and female fruits. The male eggplant is reputed to be less bitter. The male has fewer seeds and can be identified by looking at the spot on its bottom side. The round spot is male, the long spot is female. We are accustomed to seeing long eggplant with purple skin, but Chinese eggplant has beautiful white skin (which gives the vegetable its name) and is tastier. A round, Italian eggplant with purple skin that lightens to pink near the stem has become available at markets lately, and is excellent.

Eggplant Curry

- 1 ½ cups chopped onion
- 2 cloves garlic, minced
- 1 tsp cayenne
- 1 tsp cumin
- 1 medium eggplant, unpeeled, cut into 1-inch cubes and drained (see Eggplant)
- 1 ½ cups sweet peas, steamed (or ½ cup each chopped broccoli, diced carrots, diced celery, etc.)
- 1 T fresh coriander leaves (Parsley) chopped
- 1 tsp turmeric

Sauté onion, turmeric, cayenne, and cumin in a large, heavy skillet until onion is translucent. Add eggplant. Sauté, covering well with the spice mixture. Cover and cook, stirring often, for about 15 minutes. Eggplant cubes should be tender, but not mushy. A little additional water may be added if mixture is too dry.

Add ½ of the fresh coriander and cook 2 minutes longer. Serve immediately, topped with coriander and the vegetable(s).

OPTIONAL: 1 large tomato, peeled and chopped can be added at this point.

Serves 4

Eggplant Parmigiana

1 sautéed eggplant
black pepper to taste
1/4 tsp dried basil
1 clove garlic, minced
1/3 cup chopped onions
2 1/2 cups plum tomatoes

Sauté garlic and onions in a tablespoon of water in a heavy skillet until onion is transparent. Add tomatoes, basil. Stir, and cook stirring occasionally for 30 minutes.

Preheat oven to 350 degrees (moderate). Alternate layers of eggplant slices and tomatoes. Bake 30 minutes. SERVES 2-3

Italian Asparagus

1 lb fresh cooked Asparagus
2 T chopped green onions
1 medium prepared tomato
1/8 tsp dried oregano leaves
Fresh ground black pepper to taste
1/8 tsp dried thyme leaves
2 T nutritional yeast (provides the delicious "cheesy" taste)

While asparagus is cooking, combine all ingredients in a bowl. Mix well. Arrange the cooked asparagus on a serving platter. Spoon tomato mixture over asparagus.

Kale Greens

1 bunch kale greens
2 cups water
1 medium pot

Remove stem from greens, wash and rinse 3-4 times. Once clean, place greens into pot with the 2 cups water. Bring to boil, reduce heat to medium for 10-15 min. Once tender (but still slightly crisp) remove from pot and enjoy.

Mushrooms

¼ lb mushrooms per person

Wipe mushrooms with a damp cloth. Do not wash unless they are sandy. Trim the stems and slice or chop. Toss mushroom slices in a tablespoon of water over medium heat. Stir frequently to turn while sautéing. Mushrooms are done in 2-3 minutes.

Prepared Tomatoes

When recipes call for tomatoes, it's relatively easy to use fresh ones. Boil a pot of water. Add fresh, whole tomatoes and boil about 30 seconds. Remove with a slotted spoon or tongs. With a sharp knife, cut out the stem end, and from that end, peel the skin off the tomato. It will come away easily. Holding the tomato in your hand, palm down above a bowl, gently squeeze the tomato to release the seeds and some of the water. (Tomatoes add thickening to recipes, so the less juice the better.) Discard the juice, skin, and seeds. Chop tomatoes coarsely and add to soups, stews, sauces, etc.

Ratatouille

1 small eggplant
1 large onion, sliced thinly
5 ripe plum tomatoes
Black pepper to taste
3 cloves garlic, minced
1 T capers
½ cup sliced black olives
½ tsp dried oregano or ¼ tsp dried basil

To prepare: Slice the zucchini. Peel and cube eggplant. Drain for 1 hour. Prepare the tomatoes.

Use a large skillet with a cover to sauté onion and garlic in water, until onion is translucent. Add the zucchini, eggplant cubes, olives, and green pepper to the skillet. Season with basil or oregano, and pepper. Cover and cook slowly for an hour.

Add the tomatoes. Simmer uncovered until the mixture has thickened. Add capers during last 15 minutes of cooking.

Serve hot a vegetable side dish, or cold as an appetizer.

Sautéed Eggplant

1 eggplant
1 clove garlic, minced
½ tsp dried oregano or ¼ tsp dried basil
1 onion, sliced
1 T chopped fresh parsley

Peel eggplant. Drain (see Eggplant, above). Slice into ½-inch pieces crosswise. Seasoned with parsley and basil or oregano. Sauté onion and garlic in waterless cookware or steam until onion is translucent. When water is hot, add eggplant slices. Sauté for about 4 minutes on a side or until tender. Add water if needed. Serve hot. SERVES 4

Sautéed Spinach

Cooked spinach, see above
1 clove garlic, minced
3 scallions

Cook spinach about 2 minutes. Remove spinach to a bowl and squeeze excess moisture out (if spinach is too hot, use the back of a wooden spoon). Chop spinach coarsely. Wash scallions well. Trim roots and tops of stalks. Slice into ¼-inch rounds crosswise. Add scallions and garlic. Sauté 1 minute. Add spinach. Continue sautéing, constantly stirring over medium-low heat for 3 minutes.

Make extra Sautéed Spinach and refrigerate to use later in an omelet. SERVES 4

Snow Pea Pods

Snow peas are expensive, but when used as flavoring a little goes a long way. Trim the ends. They require very little cooking and are delicious raw in salads or by themselves. Sauté in water for a minute or two. In sautéed dishes, add snow pea pods at the end and cook for a minute or so. In steamed vegetable medleys and wok cooking, add snow pea pods about a minute before dish is finished cooking.

Spinach

2 lbs spinach

Spinach is grown in sandy soil and must be washed very well to get the grit out. Trim off the stem ends of the spinach with a sharp knife. Fill a large bowl with water. Soak the spinach in water. Lift the spinach out of the water into a colander. Pour the water out. Repeat the process until the sand is washed away. (Use clean water to rinse — if you pour the soaking water over the spinach, you will just pour the sand back over the spinach in the process.) Pick over the leaves, discarding those that are bruised. Cut off stems. Use a large saucepan to steam or waterless cook spinach. Pack spinach in. It will wilt down to about 1/5 the original volume when cooked. Cook about 4 minutes. SERVES 4

Stuffed Eggplant

2 lbs eggplant
½ cup vegetable broth (see page 40)
4 ounces rice pilaf
1 tsp onion, minced
4 Brazil nuts, chopped
1/4 tsp ground black pepper
1/4 cup chopped mushrooms
1 T chopped parsley

Slice the top off the eggplant, right under the leafy green cap. Follow the lines of the cap to create a scalloped edge. Save the top for a lid. Scoop out the pulp, leaving a ½-inch shell. Add the pulp to a small quantity of boiling water or stock. Cook until tender and drain.

In a large bowl, combine the cooked pulp with the remainder of the ingredients. Preheat the oven to 400 degrees. Fill the shell. Cover with the leaf lid. Bake eggplant until filling is heated (about 45 minutes to an hour).

ALTERNATE RECIPE: Bring a kettle of water to a boil. Drop eggplant in and boil 15 minutes, covered. Remove from water. Drain and slice eggplant in half lengthwise. Carefully remove pulp, leaving ½-inch shell.

Chop the eggplant pulp and add it to the stuffing ingredients above. Fill each eggplant shell half with stuffing. Place on baking pan and bake at 350 degrees, about 45 minutes. Serve as-is, or top with tomato sauce.

Stuffed Green Peppers

6 large green peppers
2 cup rice pilaf
½ cup onion, chopped
3 T chopped parsley or coriander
1 clove garlic, minced
¾ lb Portobello mushrooms
freshly ground black pepper
¾ cup vegetable broth or tomato juice (homemade or low sodium)

Trim the stem ends from the peppers and carefully remove seeds and pith.

In a large skillet, sauté onion and garlic until onion is translucent. Add mushrooms, stirring until browned. Stir in rice, parsley, and pepper. Mix well. Set aside until the mixture is cool enough to work with. When cool, stuff peppers with mixture.

Place the stuffed peppers in a baking dish. Pour broth or juice over and around them. Bake until the peppers are tender, 30-40 minutes at 350 degrees. Baste occasionally with pan liquid, adding more liquid if necessary.

Stuffed Zucchini

2 large zucchini
Stuffed eggplant stuffing
1 clove garlic, crushed or minced
8 T tomato sauce, homemade or low sodium

Wash zucchini thoroughly. Do not trim the ends. Steam whole zucchini for 2 minutes. Remove from heat. Slice in half lengthwise. Scoop out meat of zucchini leaving ¼-inch-thick shell. Prepare stuffing for stuffed eggplant, replacing the eggplant meat with the zucchini meat.

Place the stuffed zucchini in a baking pan and add garlic. Cover and bake at 350 degrees until tender, 40-45 minutes. Remove from pan. Garnish with heated tomato sauce.

SERVES 4

Tomatoes

Tomatoes can be a wonderful fruit (although we call them vegetables) when eaten freshly picked, ripe, and organically grown. In that condition, they contain vitamins A, B-complex, and important minerals. They usually retain much of their nutrients for 5-6 days after picking, under refrigeration. Tomatoes can be ripened upside down on a windowsill for a few days, but will never taste as good as vine-ripened ones. Unfortunately, most of those fresh red tomatoes in the supermarket were grown without minerals, picked green weeks ago, ripened in transit with ethylene gas, and taste like cardboard. Organically grown canned tomatoes, unsalted, are a good alternative. Commercially canned tomatoes, although possibly packed when fresh, often contain salt, sugar and other chemicals. Fresh tomatoes cannot be frozen. Italian plum tomatoes are generally sweeter. Hothouse and hydroponic tomatoes available off season are usually inferior, unless organically grown.

Zucchini

1 small zucchini per person

Zucchini is very alkalinizing and is a useful balance to the more acidic animal protein. Wash zucchini well. Trim ends. Slice in ¼-inch crosswise pieces (or julienne). Steam or waterless cook for 5 minutes. Serve with lemon juice.

SOUPS

Black Bean Soup

1 lb black (turtle) beans
2 T finely chopped parsley
1 medium carrot
2 minced garlic
1 ½ cup puréed Prepared Tomatoes
1 tsp sweet basil
2 medium onions, finely chopped
2 stalks celery, finely chopped
1 T seasoning (Cajun, curry, or Mrs. Dash)
Lime (or lemon)

Pick over and wash beans. Put in a large pot. Cover generously with water and let soak overnight or all day. Add water. Bring beans to a boil and simmer very gently, covered, about 1 1/2 hours until soft but not mushy.

Add carrots, onions, celery, garlic, parsley, tomato purée, basil, and seasonings. Simmer another ½ hour until vegetables lose most of their crunch.

Broccoli Soup w/Red Bell Pepper Creamer

Yields: serves 4
1 cup chopped broccoli
1 cup spinach, collards, or kale
2 cups water
1/2 tsp lime zest
1 cup cashews (soaked for 1 hour prior to using)

Place all ingredients into a food processor and blend until very smooth.

Red Bell Pepper Creamer

Yields: 1 cup
½ cup cashews (soaked for 1 hour prior to using)
1 cup red bell pepper, seeded and finely chopped
1 T lime juice
½ tsp lime zest
2-3 T pure water, not tap

Blend all ingredients until smooth. Pour a cup of broccoli soup into a bowl and add a tablespoon or more of Red Bell Pepper Creamer on top of the soup.

Citrus Gazpacho

2-3 grapefruits
2 tomatoes, chopped
1 small cucumber, seeded, peeled, chopped
1 small shallot, finely chopped
½ green pepper, finely chopped
1-2 cloves garlic, minced
1 T snipped fresh basil or 1 tsp dried basil
8 ounces tomato juice, homemade or low sodium
1-2 T red wine or balsamic vinegar
1/8 tsp cayenne pepper

Peel the grapefruits with a knife removing skin and pith. Working over a bowl, cut out sections, then squeeze all juice out of what remains. With scissors or a knife, cut sections into bite-size pieces. Add remaining ingredients. Stir well and chill at least 2 hours, or overnight if possible.

TO SERVE: garnish with additional basil or chopped green onions

Cold Green Kale Soup

1 cup freshly squeezed orange juice
¼ cup water
½ apple, chopped (not necessarily peeled)
¼ cup fresh basil (dill or cilantro are options)
1 clove garlic
½ green onion, chopped
1 medium cucumber, chopped
A pinch cayenne pepper
1-2 T freshly squeezed lemon juice
1 mango, peeled and chopped
4 cup kale, chopped and packed (collards work too, or any greens)

Combine water, orange juice, apple, basil, lemon, garlic, green onions, cucumber, and cayenne pepper in a strong food processor and blend. Add kale slowly and keep processing. Add mango and process until smooth. Serve in small bowls and enjoy every bite!

Gazpacho

1 clove garlic, peeled
1 red onion, sliced
1/8 tsp cayenne
1 cucumber sliced, seeded
¼ cup vinegar
3 Prepared Tomatoes
1 green pepper, seeded
¾ cup tomato juice
1 T hot pepper, chopped
2 T lemon or lime juice

Purée garlic, onion, cucumber, tomatoes, green pepper, and hot pepper in blender, food processor, or sieve vegetables and mix well with vegetable broth. Season with cayenne, vinegar, tomato and lemon juice. Chill about 3 hours, along with olives, soup tureen and soup bowls. Gazpacho must be served ice-cold.
SERVES 8

Garnish I

1 can ripe olives, sliced
1 onion, chopped
1 green pepper, chopped
1 clove garlic
1 diced cucumber

Portion out chopped fresh tomato, cucumber, onion, green pepper and pimento in separate bowls. Pour chilled liquid in each bowl. Top with sliced olives and/or croutons.

Rosemary Red Lentil Soup

Makes 12 cups

This is a very pretty soup with the red lentils, bits of tomato, and all of the greens. The mint and dill combine into a really good flavor. If you don't have fresh mint, use 1 tsp of dried mint.

- 12 cloves garlic, chopped well
- 8 green onions, chopped
- 1 15-ounce can diced no salt tomatoes
- ¼ cup fresh mint, chopped
- 1 tsp dried oregano
- 2 cups red lentils
- 8 sprigs fresh rosemary, chopped
- 7 cup broth or water
- 12 ounce fresh spinach or any greens
- 1 tsp pepper
- 3 T lemon juice and the zest

In a soup pot stir-fry garlic and green onions in water, wine, vegetable broth, etc. for about 2 minutes until the greens begin to wilt. Add diced tomatoes, mint, and oregano and cook, stirring often for two minutes more. Add lentils, broth or water and bring to a boil. Cover, turn the heat to low and simmer until the lentils are tender but not mushy (about 15 minutes). Stir in dill, spinach, pepper, lemon zest and juice and cook another few minutes.

Spicy Vegetable Broth

Vegetable broth can be made from any mixture of leaves and parts of vegetables that you would normally throw away, such as bruised lettuce leaves, potato skins, and carrot tops. When preparing salads and vegetables for steaming, save the discards for 2-3 days until you have enough for soup. Experiment to find flavors you like with different combinations of vegetables and different combinations of herbs.

    1 onion studded with cloves
    ½ lb spinach
    2 carrots
    3-4 sprigs parsley
    2 stalks celery
    kale
    1-2 cloves garlic
    1 tsp cayenne
    herb bouquet (thyme, sage)

Trim onion, leaving skin on, stud with cloves. Trim carrots and peel or scrape skin, cut into 2-inch pieces. Trim celery and remove leaves. Cut each stalk into 3 pieces. Garlic can be cooked with skin on. Wash parsley. Trim kale. For the purposes of vegetable broth, stalks can be left on spinach and kale. Carrot tops are also a good broth ingredient.

Spicy Vegetable Broth (sometimes called potassium broth, when used in juice fasts) makes an excellent, refreshing, and restorative drink, hot or cold. It will keep several days in the refrigerator. It can also be frozen for later use as a base for more complex soups, flavoring in stews, rice or other grains, etc.

Split Pea Soup

3 cups dry split peas
8 cups water
1 bay leaf
1 tsp dry mustard
1 large onion, chopped (about 1 cup)
4-5 medium garlic cloves (crushed)
3 ribs celery, finely chopped (about ¾ cup)
3 medium carrots, sliced or diced
2 medium sweet potatoes, sliced, then cut like French fries
Freshly ground black pepper
3-4 T red wine or balsamic vinegar
1 large ripe tomato, diced (about 1 cup)
lots of chopped cilantro or parsley

Place split peas, water, bay leaf, and mustard in a heavy soup pot. Bring to a boil, lower heat and simmer partially for about 20 minutes. Add onions, garlic, celery, carrots, and sweet potatoes. Cover and simmer for about 40 minutes, stirring occasionally. Add water if soup seems too thick. Add black pepper and vinegar to taste and serve topped with diced tomatoes and cilantro or parsley.

Sweet Potato Red Lentil Soup with Greens

Serves 8-10
2 large onions, chopped
1 tsp ground cumin
2 T fresh ginger, chopped
8 cup vegetable broth or low sodium broth
2 large sweet potatoes, cubed, not necessary to peel (about 4 cups)
1 1/3 cups red lentils
1 bunch (6 cups) Swiss chard, spinach, kale or collards (spine removed on kale and collards) and cut into bite-size pieces
2-4 tsp lemon juice and zest
½ tsp pepper, ground

Stir-fry onions in a large soup pot over medium heat until soft. Add water or broth as necessary to avoid burning. Stir in cumin and ginger and continue stir-frying until well mixed. Add the broth, sweet potatoes, and lentils to the onions. Bring to a boil, then turn the heat down and simmer uncovered for 30 minutes until sweet potatoes are soft and lentils are tender. Blend in batches in a food processor or use an immersion blender right in the pot until soup is creamy. Steam or lightly bake kale or collard greens until soft. Drain and add to the soup. They stay very green this way. (If using spinach or Swiss chard, add directly to the pot just before lemon and pepper. They melt quickly.) Add lemon juice, zest and pepper.

Tomato Soup

Yields: 1 ½ - 2 cups
½ cup water
½ tsp crushed fresh garlic or powdered garlic
¼ tsp onion powder
½ tsp zest of a lime
1 ripe red tomato, seeded and chopped (about 1 ¾ cups)
1 tsp minced basil, fresh or dried

Place all the ingredients into a food processor. Blend well, serve immediately.

Tofu Broth

4-5 lb extra-firm tofu
1 T dill weed
1 large onion with skin (for color)
2-5 whole cloves
1-2 stalks celery
1-2 carrots
1-2 sprigs parsley
1 tsp thyme
½ tsp rosemary
black pepper
¼ tsp turmeric (for color)

Herb bouquet: Lay out a damp piece of cheesecloth. Place parsley on it. Sprinkle with dill, thyme, rosemary, and sage. Wrap cloth around parsley and herbs. Tie with kitchen string. Or add all herbs directly to the boiling water.

Place extra firm tofu in large kettle, Dutch oven or stock pot. Cover with water. Bring to a boil.

While water is heating, prepare vegetables. Cut ends off onion, but leave skin on for color. Stud onion with 2-5 cloves (that is, insert clove by piercing the onion's flesh with the pointed end of the clove). Trim ends and leaves off 1-2 celery stalks. Trim washed carrots and cut into three pieces crosswise.

Allow water to boil for a few minutes. Skim scum from surface of soup with slotted spoon or cheesecloth. Repeat several times. Then add all the vegetables and seasonings.

Cover pot. Lower heat so soup just simmers. Simmer 1 hour. Soup can be used at this point. Remove vegetables with slotted spoon and discard.

Strain soup through fine sieve, strainer or cheesecloth. Serve plain or as:

TOFU BROTH WITH RICE: add ½ cup Rice Pilaf.

TRADITIONAL: As a main course, serve the freshly cooked hot soup. Remove vegetables. Add fresh carrot and onion slices and simmer about 10 minutes.

STORAGE AND SERVING: If hot soup is poured into canning jars and the lids are secured immediately, it can be kept up to 3 weeks in unopened jars in the refrigerator. Soup can also be frozen in plastic ½-pint containers for later use in other recipes.

Tofu Vegetable Soup

4 cups Tofu Broth (above)
4-5 Prepared Tomatoes
5-6 chopped mushrooms with stems
1 cup diced zucchini
1 tsp dried basil
1 stalk celery
1 tsp paprika
1 cup Extra Firm Tofu
2 cloves garlic, minced
½ cup chopped onion
2 diced carrots
freshly ground black pepper

Combine 1 cup tofu broth, tomatoes, and herbs in a 6 quart saucepan, stockpot, or Dutch oven. Bring to a boil and simmer 10 minutes. Meanwhile, in a large skillet sauté vegetables for 4-5 minutes. Add the vegetables, 3 more cups of broth, and pepper and simmer uncovered to 10 additional minutes. Serve hot. SERVES 6-8

Vegetable Broth

1 T dill weed
¼ tsp turmeric
1 large onion with skin (for color)
1 tsp thyme
½ tsp sage
2-5 whole cloves
½ tsp rosemary
1-2 stalks celery
1-2 carrots
Black pepper
1-2 sprigs parsley

Herb bouquet: Lay out a damp piece of cheesecloth. Place parsley on it. Sprinkle with dill, thyme, rosemary, and sage. Wrap cloth around parsley and herbs. Tie with kitchen string. Or add all herbs directly to the boiling water.

Place extra firm tofu in large kettle, Dutch oven or stock pot. Cover with water. Bring to a boil.

While water is heating, prepare vegetables. Cut ends off onion, but leaving skin on for color. Stud onion with 2-5 cloves (that is, insert clove by piercing the onion flesh with the pointed end of the clove). Trim ends and leaves off 1-2 celery stalks. Trim washed carrots and cut three pieces crosswise.

Allow water to boil for a few minutes. Skim scum from surface of soup with slotted spoon of cheesecloth. Repeat several times. Then add all the vegetables and seasonings.

Cover pot. Lower heat so soup just simmers. Simmer 1 hour. Soup can be used at this point. Remove vegetables with slotted spoon and discard.

Vegetable Soup

5-6 chopped mushrooms with stems
4-5 Prepared Tomatoes
1 cup diced zucchini
1 tsp dried basil
1 stalk celery, diced
1 tsp paprika
3 cups vegetable broth
2 cloves minced garlic
½ cup chopped onion
freshly ground black pepper
2 diced carrots

Combine broth, tomatoes, and herbs in a 6 quart saucepan, stockpot, or Dutch oven. Bring to a boil and simmer for 10 minutes. Meanwhile, sauté the vegetables for 4-5 minutes. Add the vegetables, pepper, and simmer uncovered for 10 more minutes. Serve hot. Serves 6-8

STORAGE AND SERVING: If hot soup is poured into canning jars and the lids are secured immediately, it can be kept up to 3 weeks in unopened jars in the refrigerator. Soup can also be frozen in plastic, ½ pint containers for later use in other recipes.

TRADITIONAL USE: As a main course, serve the freshly cooked hot soup. Remove vegetables. Add fresh carrot and onion slices and simmer about 10 minutes.

Vegetable Kale Soup

Yields: 3 cups/3 servings
1 small spoigani squash, chopped (about 1 ½ cups)
1 cup water
1 ripe tomato, seeded and not chopped
1 green onion, chopped
1 celery stalk, chopped fine
1 tsp crushed garlic (1 clove)
1 tsp freshly squeezed lemon juice
2 cups chopped kale
5 large basil leaves or 3 T dried basil
¼ tsp cayenne (optional)
1 cup chopped carrots
1 cup purple onion

Put all ingredients except kale in a blender with the "S" blade and process until smooth. Once blended and smooth, add kale, stir, and let rest for 15 minutes.

Winter Squash Soup

3 cups cubed winters squash
4 cups Vegetable Broth
1 diced onion
Cajun seasoning
½ cup sliced celery

Steam whole squash for a ½ hour on a rack over water either on the stove in a covered pot, or in the oven over a roasting pan. Remove squash, let cool enough to work with. Peel and remove seeds. Cut into 1 inch cubes (prepare ahead).
Place squash, onion, and celery in stock and simmer over low flame for ½ hour. Remove vegetables, saving soup. Mash vegetables

or process lightly in food processor or blender. Return mixture to soup. Season. Simmer 5-10 minutes longer.

SALADS

Salads have endless variety. They can be served hot or cold, or served as an appetizer, after the entrée, or as the entrée. They can be fruit and/or vegetable and are never quite the same twice.

Although iceberg or head lettuce is considered a sweet delicacy in France (because apparently the French know how to cut and serve it) there are many interesting salad greens. They may be used individually or in combination with other greens and ingredients. Leaves are best torn into bite-sized pieces. Consider: Boston, Bibb or cos lettuce, romaine, ruby or green leaf, chicory, arugula, radicchio, watercress, spinach, and beet tops. Field greens, such as dandelion (before the flowers have set) and lamb's quarters are also wonderful.

Salad ingredients should be washed and dried before use. The salad spinner is a great time-saver for this. Fill the basket with washed, shredded greens and spin the basket. The old-fashioned, low tech method is to spread out a large terrycloth towel. Place whole lettuce leaves next to each other on the towel, then roll the towel into a cylinder and pat gently. Unroll and repeat until all greens are dried.

You can make enough salad for two or three days. Without dressing the salad, store the surplus in a well-closed plastic bag from which all the air has been eliminated. Do not put salad dressing on the salad until you are ready to eat it—unless you like vinaigrette-pickled salad. In that case, the dressed salad is stored in an appropriately covered container for 3-12 hours before eating the salad. This could also be last night's leftovers for lunch.

Armenian Salad

4 large Prepared Tomatoes
2 cucumbers, diced
A pinch of basil
2 stalks celery, sliced
A pinch of dried mint or 1 tsp fresh
¼ tsp tarragon
½ cup red onion, chopped
½ bunch chopped watercress
¼ dried thyme
fresh juice of 1 lemon
¼ cup chopped parsley (or coriander)

Prepared tomatoes. If cucumbers are waxed to preserve them, peel. Otherwise, leave skin on.

Combine tomatoes, cucumbers, celery, onions, watercress, thyme, parsley, basil, and mint in a large bowl. Toss. Pour lemon juice onto salad and mix well.

Basic Tossed Salad

Salad greens (see introduction)
tomato slices (or cherry tomato halves)
Cucumber slices
radishes, diced
Mushrooms, sliced
scallions (1/8-inch crosswise rounds)
sweet green(red or yellow) pepper, in rings or diced

Determine amounts of ingredients by the size you want, the number of people eating, and your taste. Toss ingredients by hand or using spoons until well-mixed. Serve with dressing, fresh lemon juice and black pepper, or serve without dressing. Many other ingredients can be added according to what's available and your taste. Some suggestions are: Bermuda onion rings, shredded carrots, diced celery stalks, shredded red or green cabbage, alfalfa sprouts, sliced pitted olives, pimentos, and hot Tuscan peppers.

Cold Rice Salad

1 cup rice pilaf
1 stalk celery
¼ raw onion, chopped
6 sliced black olives
½ cup cooked broccoli (or other vegetables)
4 ounces raw cashew nuts, coarsely chopped

Mix all ingredients in a bowl.

Cole Slaw

bean sprouts
Vegan mayo (See page 76)
Small head of cabbage (red and/or green)

Remove the outer leaves and core from the cabbage. Shred or chop the remaining cabbage, preparing only what you will eat now.

VARIATIONS:
1.) Use Chinese celery or bok choy
2.) add pared, diced apple or pineapple.

20-Minute Black Bean Salad

½ lime and zest
1 very large tomato, chopped
1 package organic frozen corn
½ Vidalia onion, chopped
1 bunch cilantro, chopped
3 T balsamic vinegar or more to taste
2 cans black beans drained and rinsed **WELL!**
1 can sliced water chestnuts, drained and rinsed

Add beans, tomatoes, corn, onions, and water chestnuts to a bowl and mix. (Rinsing the beans well keeps the salad from looking grey.) Add cilantro, lime, and balsamic vinegar and mix again. Serve alone or with cucumber as an open-faced sandwich.

Garden Salad

2/3 cup romaine lettuce torn in pieces
3 sliced mushrooms
½ cup raw zucchini
4 cucumber slices
½ cup raw grated carrot
2 scooped avocados
¼ cup alfalfa sprouts
raw cashews to taste

Whether you are serving this salad as an entrée for 1 person or as a side salad for 2 or more will determine the size of your serving dish. Toss lettuce, zucchini, and carrot in a large salad bowl. Garnish with the remaining ingredients. Serve with Herb Dressing.

Greek Salad

Prepare the Armenian Salad. Sprinkle with sliced olives. Dress with lemon juice to taste. Sprinkle with fresh ground black pepper as desired.

Hearts of Palm Salad

Chilled, canned hearts of palm
paprika
Romaine leaf, washed, whole
stuffed olives, sliced
Green and red pepper rings
chopped parsley

Cut palms lengthwise in strips. Serve over bed romaine lettuce. Garnish with pepper rings and olives.

Hummus

1 8-oz can chickpeas, rinsed and drained
¼ cup red bell pepper, diced
1 T lemon juice
1 tsp garlic, finely chopped
Freshly ground black pepper

Easy to make. Purée chickpeas in a blender with lemon juice, red bell pepper, and garlic until they become creamy and thick. Add pepper to taste. Serve with pita bread. SERVES 8

Mock Tuna Salad

Chef's notes: 1 small dill pickle may be shredded or minced and used in place of the relish. You can also add a light squirt of lemon juice for added flavor.

15 ounces chickpeas, drained and rinsed
¼ cup red onion, chopped
2 whole celery stalks
2 tsp nutritional yeast (optional)
2 T relish (dill pickle) unsweetened
2 T vegan mayo (fat-free) (See page 76)
½ tsp kelp

In a large mixing bowl, mash chickpeas with a fork until coarse and no whole beans are left. Alternatively, pulse beans in a food processor a few times—be careful not to purée them—and transfer to a mixing bowl. Shred celery with cheese grater or pulse a few times in food processor. Transfer to the mixing bowl and add remaining ingredients, stirring to combine. Add more vegan mayo and/or kelp as necessary or desired and black pepper to taste.

Salad Nicoise

1 clove garlic
2 peeled, quartered tomatoes
12 coarsely chopped pitted black olives
1 cucumber peeled, finely chopped
1 cup Romaine lettuce, torn in pieces

Rub salad bowl with garlic. Add all ingredients and toss well.

Special Green Salad

Romaine
tomatoes, chopped
Cucumbers, sliced/halved
broccoli cut into ½-inch pieces
Kale, collards or Swiss chard, stems removed (except Swiss chard) and cut into 2-inch pieces
1 can black beans, drained and rinsed

Combine lettuce of choice, tomatoes, and cucumber in a large bowl. Put 2 inches of water in a large saucepan, bring to a boil, add broccoli and kale or greens of choice, cover and cook about 4 minutes or until greens are tender and broccoli is just soft. Drain well and allow to cool a little while making dressing. Add beans and broccoli, greens and salad dressing. Mix well and your meal in one bowl is ready to go.

Spring Salad Mix

Yields: serve 2
1 bunch red leaf lettuce cut or torn into small pieces
½ cup green cabbage, chopped fine
1 tomato diced (1 cup)
½ purple onion, chopped (about ½ cup)
½ red bell pepper cut into thin strips

In a large bowl, combine the ingredients (except tomato). Toss until well mixed. Add tomato just before serving.

Strawberry-Spinach Salad

1 tsp poppy seeds
2 cups sliced fresh strawberries
¼ cup freshly squeezed orange juice
½ lb fresh spinach, washed, trimmed and torn

DRESSING: Combine orange juice and poppy seeds in small bowl. Stir well.
SALAD: Wash spinach, trim and tear leaves. Toss spinach and strawberries in a large bowl. Arrange on individual salad plates. Drizzle the dressing over each salad. SERVES 6-8

Tangy Lime Cole Slaw

Serves 6
Cole Slaw:
½ medium cabbage, cored and finely shredded
2 carrots, peeled and shredded
¼ medium red cabbage, cored and finely shredded

Tangy Lime Dressing:
½ cup Vegan mayo
¼ cup water
2 limes, zest and juice
2 garlic cloves, minced
½-1 tsp jalapeño pepper, remove seeds and mince

Toss the cabbage and carrots in a large bowl. Combine the mayonnaise, water, lime juice, lime zest, garlic, and jalapeño in a blender and process until smooth.

Adjust jalapeños to desired spiciness. Pour the dressing over the vegetables before serving and toss well.

Tomato Salad

2 large tomatoes
black olives, organic, pitted and chopped
Balsamic (sugar free) vinegar
capers

Slice tomatoes. Arrange on 4 salad plates. Drizzle 1 tsp balsamic vinegar over each serving. Sprinkle olives and capers.

Tomato Salad with Turkish Tahini Dressing

Yields: Serves 4-6 (the recipe makes ½ cup dressing)
1 ½ lbs tomatoes, green and/or red, cored and sliced
4 T sesame tahini
1/2 tsp cumin seeds, lightly toasted and ground
1/3 cup water
2 T freshly squeezed lemon juice
1-2 cloves garlic
1-2 T flat leaf parsley, chopped
Freshly ground pepper

Arrange tomatoes on a platter. Combine tahini, water and lemon juice. In a mortar and pestle mash garlic to a paste. Stir into the tahini mixture. Add cumin and pepper to taste. Thin with water if the dressing is too thick to pour. Drizzle over the sliced tomatoes, sprinkle on the parsley, and serve.

ADVANCED PREPARATION: The dressing is good for a couple of days in the refrigerator, but will thicken and become more pungent. Thin out with water if desired.

DISHES

Black Bean Brownies

½ cup Cacao powder (raw chocolate powder)
1 15-ounce can black beans, rinsed and drained
1 ½ cup date syrup
2 T flax seeds
1 tsp baking powder
½ tsp baking soda
3 tsp vanilla extract (no-alcohol vanilla extract)
¾ cup barley flour or whole wheat pastry flour
½ cup vegan chocolate chips (optional)

In a food processor, blend all ingredients except vegan chocolate chips. Blend well approximately 1 minute. Add vegan chocolate chips. Put in an 8 x 8 glass baking dish or silicone dish. Bake 25-35 minutes. Brownies should have movement. Cool 10-15 minutes… Enjoy!

Black Beans and Rice

Brown rice (long or short grained)
chopped tomatoes
chopped red, yellow or green peppers
carrots (grated or julienned)
water chestnuts
cilantro, chopped
Frozen corn, thawed
arugula, chopped
1 can black beans, rinse and add back a little water
Low sodium tamari or Braggs Liquid Aminos
salsa
Chopped Vidalia, green onions, red onions or some of each

Cook rice. Heat beans. Put all chopped vegetables in individual dishes. Start your plate with rice, then beans, and just pile it up high and top it all with low sodium tamari. The tamari is the secret for making it delicious, but if you prefer salsa, use that.

Cuban Black Beans Over Rice

2 15-ounce cans black beans, drained and rinsed
1 ½ cup water
1 large onion, chopped
2 green peppers, chopped
1 red bell pepper, chopped
1 clove garlic, chopped
3 bay leaves
½ tsp cumin
1 cup cooked brown rice

Sauté the onions, green and red peppers and garlic in water until translucent. Combine all ingredients. Cook on stove with low heat until beans are tender and the liquid has thickened. Serve over brown rice with raw chopped onions.

Chickpeas, Cinnamon, Cumin, and Carrots

Serves 4
1 large onion, thinly sliced and halved
¼ cup dried currents
3 medium carrots, sliced into thin rounds
1 tsp turmeric
2 cup water or vegetable broth
1 tsp ground cinnamon
2 14.5-ounce cans chick peas, rinsed and drained
¼ cup (or more) parsley or cilantro
3 cloves garlic, chopped (1 T)
1 tsp cumin
¼ tsp cayenne pepper
pepper to taste

Stir fry onions over medium heat until soft. Add garlic and cook a minute more. Add vegetable broth, chickpeas, carrots, currents, turmeric, cinnamon, cumin, cayenne, and stir. Add pepper and parsley.

Collard Sushi with Red Pepper and Cucumber

Substitute cooked asparagus or green beans, long carrot or bok choy strips, cooked greens, rice, beans, etc., for the filling. They make perfect sushi like hors d'oeuvres, or use instead of sandwiches.

1 bunch collard greens
2 green onions, chopped
8 T hummus made without tahini or oil
½ cup cilantro, chopped
¼ red pepper, cut in thin strips
¼ cup shredded carrots
¼ small cucumber, cut in thin strips (skin optional)
½ lemon

Put about 2 inches of water in a large frying pan and bring to a boil. Choose 4 of the finest collard greens. Lay them flat, cut off the thick stem at the point where the leaf begins, then pile them on top of each other in the boiling water. Cover and cook for about 30 seconds to a minute. Collards are pretty tough and don't easily break apart when cooked. Their flexibility makes them a perfect wrap. Drain, then lay flat on a board or counter with the thick part of the stem facing up. Down the center spine of each collard leaf place a row of about 2 T hummus, sprinkle with green onions, cilantro and shredded carrots. Place thin red pepper strips and cucumber strips on top. Start with the side nearest you, flip it over and gently roll into a sausage shape. With a sharp knife, cut into as many small pieces as possible. Yields six or more depending on size of collard greens.

Chili Bean Cornbread Casserole

Chili Bean Filling:
1 T unsweetened applesauce
3 cloves garlic, minced
1 medium yellow onion, diced
1 cup corn, fresh or frozen
2 tsp chili powder
1 tsp ground cumin
1 tsp dried oregano
15-ounce tomato sauce
15-ounce pinto beans, drained and rinsed
1 T tamari
2 T Mrs. Dash (original)
15-ounce kidney beans, drained and rinsed
1 tsp black pepper
1 T Bragg's Liquid Aminos or coconut Aminos
1 medium bell pepper, diced and seeded

Cornbread Topping:
¾ cup unsweetened almond milk
2 tsp apple cider vinegar
½ cup cornmeal
½ cup whole wheat flour
½ tsp baking soda
½ tsp baking powder
1 T unsweetened applesauce

Preheat oven to 425 degrees F. In a 12-inch sauté pan, heat applesauce over medium heat. Add garlic, onions, peppers, corn and cook until onions are translucent, about 5 minutes. Add chili powder, cumin, oregano, beans and tomato sauce, mix thoroughly and cook for an additional minute. Spread mixture evenly in a 8 x 8 glass baking dish.

In a measuring cup, mix soy milk and apple cider vinegar and set aside for 10 minutes to allow soy milk to curdle.

In a medium bowl, whisk together the cornmeal, flour, baking powder, and baking soda. Add soy milk mixture and applesauce and mix just enough to combine. Spread batter evenly on top of the chili bean mixture. Bake 25-30 minutes or until top is golden brown and toothpick comes out clean.

"Crab" Cakes (Jackfruit)

Yields: 9 cakes
1 small onion
1 20-ounce can young green jackfruit in water, rinsed and well drained
1 15-ounce can white beans, drained
2 T poultry seasoning or Old Bay Seasoning
2 large cloves garlic, pressed
2 tsp organic soy sauce
1 tsp prepared mustard
1/8 tsp turmeric powder
½ cup oatmeal (regular or quick)

Preheat oven 350 degrees. Chop the onion finely in a food processor and place it in a medium bowl. Add jackfruit to processor. Pulse until broken into rough pieces of about ½ inch. Do not grind into a paste. Add to onions. Add white beans and all remaining ingredients except oatmeal. Pulse to distribute seasonings well. Add mixture to a bowl along with oatmeal. Stir with jackfruit and onion. Line baking sheet with parchment paper or silicone mat. Scoop up approximately 1/3 cup of mixture and shape into patty. Carefully place on prepared baking sheet and repeat with remaining mixture. Bake 20 minutes.

Inspiring Green Punch

5 kale stems
3 stalks celery
1 cucumber
1 apple
1 cup water
Place all ingredients in a blender. Blend until smooth.

Lemon Kale Sandwiches

4 slices whole grain bread without oil, or Ezekiel 1 bread
1 bunch of kale, chopped in bite-sized pieces (remove thick stem) or Swiss Chard or greens choice
Hummus without tahini
green onions (1 per slice of bread)
½ bunch cilantro or parsley, chopped
zest of lemon
1 large tomato, sliced in 4 thick slices (optional)
½ lemon, center part, very thinly sliced and the ends squeezed and zested

Toast bread well. If using Mestemacher or a rye or pumpernickel, double or triple toast. Put kale in a pot with about 4 inches of water in the bottom. Bring to a boil, cover and cook kale until tender. Check frequently. Spread toast thickly with hummus, sprinkle with green onions (on the hummus), pile cilantro on top of the green onions and then place a few thinly sliced lemons on the cilantro. When kale is tender, drain well. Shake the strainer so all water is gone, sprinkle the kale in the strainer with lemon zest and remaining lemon juice. Lots of lemon makes this good! Then put a big handful of lemon filled kale on top of each piece of bread. It is delicious just like that or topped with a tomato slice.

Protein Oat Waffles/Pancakes

Makes 10 4-inch waffles

If making waffles, a good non-stick waffle iron is important. Get Hain Pure Foods Featherweight Baking Powder or your favorite sodium-free baking powder.

- 1 can cannelloni or great northern beans, drained and rinsed
- 2 ¼ cup water
- 1 ¾ cups old-fashioned oats
- 1 heaping T ground flaxseed meal
- ½ tsp baking powder
- 1-2 tsp vanilla, non-alcoholic
- 2 cups fresh strawberries

Preheat waffle iron or pancake pan. Place beans and water in a blender and blend well. Add oats, flaxseed, baking powder, vanilla and blend until completely smooth, light and foamy. For waffles, pour about 1/3 cup of batter for each 4-inch waffle into waffle iron. Close and cook for a minimum of 8 minutes.

Raw Food Lasagna

A raw food diet is a plant-based diet that promotes uncooked and unprocessed foods, such as organic fruits, vegetables, and nuts. Raw food lasagna made from fresh Italian herbs, vegetables, and nuts, and prepared without heat, is a delicious and nutritious meal that can be eaten for lunch or dinner.

Things you need:
Food processor
4 medium bowls
Spatula
medium lasagna dish (33 cm X 27 cm)

<u>Nut Cheese</u>
2 cup macadamias
1 cup pine nuts
2 T nutritional yeast
2 organic yellow peppers
2 T fresh parsley
2 T lemon juice
1 T fresh thyme
½ cup water (as needed)

Place all ingredients in food processor and blend until smooth.

<u>Walnut Meat</u>
1 ½ cup walnuts
1 cup sun-dried tomatoes
2 T dried oregano
2 T dried sage
½ tsp cayenne pepper

Place walnuts into food processor and blend until chopped crunchy, but not fine. Set aside in small bowl. Soak sun-dried tomatoes for 30 minutes and drain. Once sun-dried tomatoes are soaked and soft, place all the ingredients in food processor and blend for about 15 seconds.

<u>Tomato Sauce</u>
1 ½ cups sun-dried tomatoes (soaked for 20 minutes in 1 cup water)
2 or 3 dates
1 ½ T dried oregano
2 cloves garlic
2 T lemon juice
2 cup organic tomatoes (chopped and seeded)

Put all ingredients into food processor and blend until very smooth. Set aside in a bowl.

<u>Spinach Layer</u>
5 cup organic spinach
5 T dried oregano
5 medium zucchini

In a glass casserole dish:
Spread tomato sauce on bottom of dish evenly
Add nut cheese to each layer
Lay one layer of spinach on top of sauce
Lay each ingredient layer by layer (you should have about 3 layers of the lasagna)
Place into your dehydrator for about 2.5 hours on 110 degrees.
Once finished, remove, add more tomato sauce, serve and enjoy!

<u>REMEMBER:</u> Nuts are fattening and should be eaten in moderation.

Rice, Beans, and Greens

Serves 2

This is the meal to make when you don't want to cook. To be even faster, use Swiss chard, which cooks quickly, or spinach, which melts in a flash.

    1 bunch kale or collard greens, stems removed and chopped
    1 cup rice
    2 cup water or vegetable broth
    1 can black beans, drained and rinsed
    1 cup cilantro
    1 tomato, chopped
    1 green onion
    Salsa or low sodium tamari or Braggs Liquid Aminos (optional)

Put rice and water or broth in rice cooker and cook until done. Warm beans in a small saucepan. Add ½ cup water to heat beans, add cilantro and stir. Chop kale into bite-size pieces and put in 2 inches boiling water, cover and cook for 2-4 minutes, depending on taste. Drain. Put drained kale on plate, top with rice, beans, chopped tomato green onions and salsa or low sodium tamari. Chopped mango is also good.

Rice "Pilaf"

1 cup whole grain rice (long, short or medium grain)
3 cups water

Wash rice in strainer. Place rice in dry heavy skillet over medium heat. Stir as kernels gently toast (about 5 minutes). If "kernels" pop, heat is too high. Cool and store for later use. Or place toasted rice immediately into 3 cups of boiling water in heavy saucepan. (**OPTIONAL:** add 1 T malt vinegar] Bring to a boil. Cover. Reduce heat to very low. Let simmer covered for 45 minutes. Fluff with a fork a few minutes before completion.

A Simple Snack

1 cup carrots, cooked
1 cup celery
1 cup red bell pepper
1 cup cucumbers

Assemble into vegetable containers and enjoy to satisfy your food cravings.

Sweet Potatoes, Black Beans

2 sweet potatoes, baked
1 can black beans, drained and rinsed
cilantro
green onions, chopped
lime juice

Cut hot sweet potatoes in half, spoon on black beans, top with red pepper, cilantro, and green onions as desired. Squeeze lime over it all. Or, for a larger presentation, remove potato flesh into a bowl and top with ingredients.

Vegetable Brown Rice

1 small zucchini, minced
small red bell pepper, minced
4 cups cooked brown rice
¾ cup minced leaks
¼ cup minced cilantro or parsley

In a large mixing bowl toss all the ingredients together except brown rice. Once well mixed, add the rice to mixture and mix well. Chill before serving. SERVES 3 TO 6

Zucchini Pasta

Yields: 1 serving
1 zucchini, peeled
(tools needed for pasta: Spiralizer)

Cut zucchini into thin noodles using a Spiralizer or a vegetable peeler to create long, thin, pasta-type "noodles."

DRESSINGS, SPREADS AND SAUCES, ETC.

Awesome Vegan Ranch Dressing

½ cup Almond milk
1 tsp onion powder
½ cup Soy vegan mayonnaise (NaSoya Nayonaise)
1 tsp garlic powder
2-3 T red wine vinegar
1 T dried or fresh parsley (finely chopped)

Mix all ingredients in food processor. I use vanilla flavored soy milk. Sounds unusual, but tastes great.

This recipe tastes totally like the regular ranch dressing on shelves in supermarkets. Everybody loves it and they all want the recipe after hearing that it is vegan and so much healthier for you. Use it on salads, brown rice, baked potatoes, steamed vegetables and a little thicker (add a bit more nayonaise) as a dip for raw vegetables (omit the red wine vinegar for the vegetable dip).

Caesar Salad Dressing

15 ounces cannellini bean or any white bean, drained and rinsed
3-4 T lemon juice (about 1 lemon)
3 cloves fresh garlic
2 T capers, rinsed
2 T mustard like Dijon
2 T nutritional yeast
Pepper to taste

Put all ingredients in a food processor and blend well. Add water or broth to thin if desired, but the thicker consistency blends well into a salad.

Dijon Vinaigrette

Makes about 1 cup
This classic, French vinaigrette is a piquant dressing for greens like romaine and red leaf lettuce.

1 T shallots, finely chopped
1 T Dijon mustard
¼ cup red wine or apple cider vinegar
freshly ground pepper to taste

Whisk together shallots, mustard and vinegar. Then season to taste with pepper.

Egg Replacer

1 cup potato flour
¾ cup tapioca flour
2 tsp baking powder

Mix well, keep in air-tight jar.

1 ½ tsp of mix + 1 T water = 1 egg yolk
1 ½ tsp of mix + 2 T water = 1 whole egg

Excellent Black Bean Salsa Dip

1 can black beans, rinsed and drained
fresh cilantro
1 16-ounce jar salsa, organic or homemade
½ juicy lime
¼ lemon juice

Mix all together and put on toasted whole wheat pita or any no-fat, whole grain cracker. This is also good, if any is left over, as a topping on rice.

Fat-Free Vegan Vinaigrette Salad Dressing

¼ cup fresh squeezed orange juice(optional)
½ cup red wine vinegar
2 tsp dried mustard
pepper to taste

Whisk together all ingredients until combined fully.
Serves 4

Fresh Cherry Tomato Salsa

1 pint cherry tomatoes, quartered
1 jalapeño pepper
1 red onion, diced finely
juice from ½ lemon
¼ cup fresh cilantro, chopped

Toss the cherry tomatoes, red onion, and jalapeño together in a small bowl. Squeeze lemon juice over mixture, and stir in fresh cilantro. Refrigerate for at least 30 minutes prior to serving.

Herbal Red Wine Vinaigrette

1/3 cup red wine vinegar
1 T Dijon mustard
1 T garlic, minced
¼ tsp pepper
¼ cup freshly chopped parsley
3 T fresh basil, chopped
2 T fresh chives, chopped
2 T fresh mint, chopped

In a small bowl, combine the red wine vinegar, garlic, and pepper and whisk well to combine. Stir in the herbs. Yields: 2 cups

Hummus Carrot Salad Dressing

¼ cup carrot juice
¼ cup balsamic vinegar
2 T hummus (no oil, no tahini)
1-2 tsp mustard (Dijon or mustard of choice)

Mix all together in a small bowl and use on any greens.

Lemon Herb Dressing

Yields: 1 cup (6-7 servings)
½ cup freshly squeezed lemon juice
½ tsp crushed garlic (1 clove)
1 T fresh or dried herbs (basil, parsley, oregano, dill)
A dash of black pepper

Place all ingredients into a bowl, whisk to combine and mix well; store in a glass jar or container in the refrigerator.

Nutritional Yeast Cheese Dip/Sauce

¼ cup nutritional yeast
1 cup water
¼ cup whole wheat pastry flour
¼ tsp garlic powder
1/8 tsp dried yellow mustard powder

Mix dry ingredients, add water, whisk until clumps are gone. Put in pot and heat on medium until thick. This is a very thick sauce. Best suited for things like macaroni and cheese, etc. You can add more water if too thick. Mixing salsa with this for nacho cheese with chips is great; adding onion powder and parsley works great for use in a scalloped potato recipe.

No-Oil Balsamic Dressing

Makes 1 ¾ cups

Drizzle this tangy dressing over green salad or steamed vegetables.

2 cup boiling water
1 cup balsamic vinegar
2 T chopped, pitted dates
2 T Dijon mustard
½ tsp vegan Worcestershire sauce
3 T nutritional yeast
1 T onion powder
1 clove garlic, minced

In a medium, heatproof bowl pour water over dates and set aside to let soak until soft, 10 to 15 minutes. Reserve ¼ cup of the soaking liquid and then drain dates and transfer to a blender. Add reserved water, vinegar, Dijon, yeast, Worcestershire, onion powder and garlic. Purée until smooth.

Parmesan Cheeze

(1 = 1 pint)
1 part ground almonds
1 part nutritional yeast
Dashes of onion powder and garlic powder
Combine all ingredients in a container with lid and shake well.

Salsa Salad Dressing

2 T no-tahini hummus
2 T salsa
2 T balsamic vinegar

Mix well and serve on greens. Vary amounts according to individual taste.

Spicy Mustard Dressing

½ cup prepared spicy smooth mustard
¼ cup red wine vinegar
2-4 T date syrup

Whisk together all ingredients.

Sun-Dried Tomato Marinara Sauce

Yields: 1 Cup, 2 serving
1 ripe tomato, chopped (makes about ½ cup)
½ cup yellow or red bell pepper, chopped
1 T fresh basil, minced (1 tsp dried)
½ -1 tsp dried oregano or fresh oregano
1 tsp garlic crushed (2 cloves)
¾ cup sun-dried tomatoes, soaked about 30-45 minutes in water (not the oil-based sun-dried tomatoes)

Put all ingredients into food processor fitted with an "S" blade and process until smooth, stopping only to scrape down the sides of the bowl with a spatula.

NOTE: The sauce will keep in the refrigerator for 3 days in a sealed container.

Combine Zucchini pasta noodles and marinara sauce and enjoy.

Note: to serve warm, heat only the sauce gently for about 1 minute and toss with the pasta. Do not microwave.

Tahini Miso Sauce

¼ cup water, more to taste
1 T mellow (light) miso
1 clove garlic, finely chopped
1/3 cup tahini
1 tsp orange zest
1 tsp lemon zest
1 T parsley chopped finely

In a medium bowl, whisk together all ingredients. For a thinner sauce, add more water. SERVES 4

Tofu-Cashew Mayonnaise

Yields: 1 pint, keeps 2-3 weeks
1 12.3-ounce package firm silken tofu
½ cup raw cashews
3 T fresh-squeezed lemon juice
1 tsp prepared mustard, any variety
1/8 tsp granulated onion powder

Drain water from tofu and place it and all ingredients in a high-speed blender. Blend at highest speed until creamy and light. Seal tightly and refrigerate.

Vegan Mayonnaise

1 pkg. firm or extra firm silken tofu
1 tsp onion or garlic powder
1 tsp yellow mustard
The juice 1 fresh lemon

Purée all in food processor. Add Dijon mustard for a great dipping sauce for artichokes or asparagus, or as a sandwich spread.

Vegan Thousand Island Salad Dressing

1 cup vegan mayonnaise
1/3 cup ketchup (low salt organic)
½ tsp onion powder
3 T dill pickle relish organic, no sugar

Whisk together all ingredients in a bowl until smooth and creamy.

RAITAS

A raitas is an Indian dish usually served as a cooling accompaniment to the spiciness of curries, but it is delicious with many western foods.

Carrot Raita

½ cup grated carrots
3 tsp dates chopped
½ tsp cayenne pepper

Wash, scrape, grate carrot. Combine all ingredients. May be chilled. SERVES 4

Cucumber Raita

1 cucumber
¾ tsp ground cumin
Dash cayenne pepper

Peel the cucumber and finely chop. Add rest of the ingredients and mix well. May be chilled. (Note: if using fresh cumin, the taste is released by roasting gently on an ungreased pan under the broiler for 5 minutes. Grind with a mortar and pestle or a spice grinder.)
SERVES 6

Banana Raita

2 ripe bananas
dash cinnamon
dash cardamom
1 tsp fresh lemon juice
dash cayenne pepper

Purée one banana in a blender or food processor (or mash by hand). Chop the other banana into ½-inch cubes. Combine all ingredients. May be chilled. SERVES 6

Watercress Raita

1 clove garlic
¼ tsp cayenne pepper
1/2 cup watercress leaves, chopped fine
1/3 sweet green pepper, chopped fine

Combine all ingredients. Chill if desired. SERVES 4

RECIPE SUBSTITUTIONS

Just about any recipe can be adapted to be healthy, vegan, and fat-free with the right substitutions.

Egg Replacement

Replacing eggs is often the trickiest part of vegan baking.

REPLACEMENT FOR 1 WHOLE EGG	WHEN TO ADD	CAUTION	WORKS BEST
¼ C SILKEN TOFU (2 OZ)	BLEND WITH	CAN BE VERY HEAVY. DO NOT USE IN RECIPES WHERE MULTIPLE EGGS MUST BE REPLACED	IN A PINCH
½ BANANA		VERY RIPE BANANAS WILL LEAVE A HINT OF FLAVOR AND INCREASE SWEETNESS	IN FAT-FREE COOKIES, BREADS, MUFFINS, PANCAKES
¼ C APPLESAUCE	ADD WITH WET INGREDIENTS	AVOID USING MORE THAN 1 CUP TOTAL IN ANY RECIPES.	IN BREADS MUFFINS, CAKES, CUP-CAKES
1/4 C NON-DAIRY LIQUID (WATER, ALMOND MILK, SOY MILK)	BLEND WITH LIQUID OR WET INGREDIENTS	CAN BE HEAVY	IN BROWNIES
2 1/2 T GROUND FLAX SEEDS MIXED WITH 3 T WATER	ADD AS "EGG" IS CALLED FOR ORIGINALLY	ADDS AN EARTHY NUTTY TASTE. CAN PROVIDE FIRM OR CHEWY	IN CHOCOLATE RECIPES, GRANOLA BARS OATMEAL COOKIES
ENER-G EGG REPLACER	ADD AS "EGG" CALLED FOR	LEAVES CHALKY TASTE	FOR BEGINNERS

To replace egg whites: combine 1 Tablespoon agar powder dissolved into 1 T of water

Buttermilk substitution:

To replace buttermilk, combine 1 cup soy milk with 1 tsp lemon juice or apple cider vinegar. Whisk until foamy and bubbly. This soy buttermilk mixture can replace buttermilk 1:1 in any baking recipe.

Fat Replacement:

Applesauce is the most common way to replace fat (e.g., oil, butter) but beans and vegetables also work as a direct replacement.

REPLACEMENT	CAUTION	WORKS BEST
APPLESAUCE	AVOID USING MORE THAN 1 C OF APPLESAUCE IN ANY RECIPE	IN CAKES, CUPCAKES, SOME COOKIES
PURÉED BEANS	BEANS ADD FUDGY TEXTURE. BE SURE TO MATCH YOUR BEANS WITH THE COLOR OF YOUR GOODIES.	IN BROWNIES OATMEAL COOKIES
CANNED PURE PUMPKIN	ADDS A HINT OF PUMPKIN FLAVOR AND ORANGE COLOR	IN MUFFINS, CHOCOLATE TREATS, OATMEAL
SHREDDED ZUCCHINI	LOCKS IN MOISTURE	IN MUFFINS, BREADS, CHOCOLATE TREATS
VEGAN CREAM CHEESE	AVOID REPLACING MORE THAN ¼ C OF MARGARINE OR SHORTENING.	IN PASTRIES, BISCUITS(ANY TIME YOU NEED TO "CUT IN" FAT)
COLD BANANA	ADDS A HINT OF BANANA FLAVOR	IN SCONES